Don't Give Up Too Soon
10 Ways to Help You ReSET Your Energy, Mindset, Wellness & Tranquility

Written By Tinesha Boswell

Written By: Tinesha Boswell
Published By: Pen Legacy®
Editor: Laura Charles-Horne
Cover Design & Formatting By: The Liar's Craft

DISCLAIMER
Although you may find the teachings, life lessons and examples in this book to be useful, the book is sold with the understanding that neither the author nor Pen Legacy® are engaged in presenting any legal, relationship, financial, emotional, or health advice.

Any person who's experiencing financial, anxiety, depression, health, or relationship issues should consult with a licensed therapist, advisor, licensed psychologist, or any qualified professional before commencing into anything described in this book. This book's intent is to provide you with the writer's account and experience with overcoming life matters. All results will differ than yours; however, our goal is to provide you with our "take" on how to overcome and be resilient when faced with circumstances.

There are lessons in every blessing.

Library of Congress Cataloging – in- Publication Data has been applied for.
ISBN: 978-0-9600483-3-5
PRINTED IN THE UNITED STATES OF AMERICA.

ACKNOWLEDGEMENTS

I would like to take this time to thank my husband, Orlando and my children. When we met, I was an entrepreneur as a Travel Agent. He understood my goals and aspirations with business at the time. Since day 1, he has never asked me to stop doing business even when I made the wrong investment in several network marketing businesses. This book was possible because he took responsibility for all the bills, along anything that would distract me from writing this book. This wouldn't be possible if he did not believe in me and respect my goals.

I would like to thank my girlfriend Tamika Lewis for always listening to my ranting and allowing me to be me when I couldn't be me with anyone else. She has encouraged me to continue this journey of life and applauded me for my decision and keeping it moving.

I want to thank my cousin Nikia, who is an author herself, for taking the time to edit my book.

I would like to thank my mom and sister for always encouraging me to keep going and pushing me pass my excuses.

I would like to thank my publisher Charron Monaye of Pen Legacy, LLC for being patient, clear, direct, loving and insightful and pushing me to complete this project in the timeline we created. Lastly, I would like to thank my grandmother Carreather Baker for always encouraging me and letting me know that I was a queen. When I pray at night, you always tell me "Baby, it's going to be alright, just stay faithful, don't let anyone stop you and no matter what, keep pushing"! For this, I am forever grateful and wish you were here today to see how much the family has grown! RIP Mom and Grandma!

TABLE OF CONTENTS

MY WHY

Over the years, I have gone to seminars, paid for classes, joined many challenges (and created some), all in an effort to try to find myself; my goal was to find out what I considered to be my "Why".

The initial idea of this book was to specifically discuss the topic of chronic illness and how your illness does not define who you are. However, in the middle of me writing this book, I had a change of heart. In October 2018, I was attending a church event in which my pastor preached about being "complete in the Lord." I wasn't sure where he was going with it until he handed out this exercise that focused on his point: being complete in the Lord! He accompanied it with scriptures and real-life applications that really emphasized his point. After completing the exercise, I realized that as women, we often don't feel "complete" within ourselves, our lives, our jobs, and our relationships. I then decided to make the purpose of this book not just about chronic illness, but also about feeling more complete.

The exercise had us to divide into 8 teams that represented the anagram of the word COMPLETE: **C**ompassion, **O**penness, **M**otivate, **P**rayer, **L**ove, **E**nthusiastic; **T**rustworthy and **E**ver Ready.

- **Compassion** by trying to feel someone's pain even though you may be perfectly fine.

- Being **Open** minded like Samuel and David when they needed a new king.
- To **Motivate** the masses, we must first motivate ourselves; according to 2 Timothy 1:7, "God doesn't give us a spirit of fear but power, love, and self-control."
- You cannot pour from an empty cup and must embrace the inner peace that comes with **Prayer**; according to 1 John 5:14, "And this is the confidence that we have toward him, that if we ask anything according to his will, he hears us."
- **Love** ourselves as He loves us and reach out to someone and show them the same love; according to 1 John 3:16, "By this, we know love, that he laid down his life for us and we ought to lay down our lives for the brothers."
- We should be **Enthusiastic** when learning about the lord and excited to spread the gospel; according to 2 Corinthians 9:7, "each one must give as he has decided in his heart, not reluctantly or under compulsion, for God loves a cheerful giver."
- People cannot grow if they cannot find you to be **Trustworthy**; according to Proverbs 11:13, "Whoever goes about slandering reveals secrets, but he who is trustworthy in spirit keeps things covered."
- No matter how hard it gets, we should always be **Ever Ready** for the Lord; according to Galatians 6:9, "And let us not grow weary of doing good, for in due season we will reap, if we do not give us."

At that moment, I thought to myself "Oh, this is a great sermon!" I also thought to myself that I should absolutely incorporate that into my book. As I was putting the above practices in place, I made sure that I used the word "complete" and all that I learned that day into this book. I also strived to use these principles to my personal and professional life.

It got my mind thinking... why? Why do we need to feel complete? In my years of experience as a Wellness Coach, I find that people see the word "complete" and think of the word "accomplishment". The church event helped me to see this issue in a new way, and it helped me to recreate the meaning and purpose of this book.

The Journey Starts Today!

I have struggled with chronic illness since the age of Three. I was diagnosed with Asthma that eventually grew into Bronchial Chronic Asthma. My first home was the hospital and then I lived with my parents. I remember being in the hospital, walking around with an IV, going into other kid's rooms giving them encouragement and letting them know that everything would be okay, that they didn't have to allow their sicknesses to keep them down. I learned that from my mom and my primary care physician, Dr. Joanna Firth. I remember Dr. Firth having a conversation with my mother saying it was okay to allow me to run, play outside, and do everything all the other children are doing because that would be the only way that I learn my own limitations. Dr. Firth also told my mom that if she stops me from being an active person, that it would affect my confidence. The doctor expressed that the goal is to build my confidence by allowing me to work through my own obstacles. As I grew older, my asthma got so bad that my doctor used to joke and say that I needed to live in an incubator because I was allergic to so many things.

It was kind of fun being in the hospital as a child because everyone loved me. The nurses would bring me food, watch tv with me, and play games when the other kids were too ill to play. As I grew older, it became less and less fun. The doctors and nurses may have shown compassion, but not middle school and high school students.

Fast forward to 1997, I have been a mom for three years and I just purchased my first home. I have been suffering with chronic asthma for 20+ years. Instead of staying home from school, I now have to call out of work because I had an asthma attack. It is not fun being an adult with a family, a car note, car insurance, medical expenses, and half a paycheck because you were ill. While all of these should have made me try to figure out a better way of living, I allowed it to affect my thought process. Was this what I had to look forward to in life? Will I always be an inpatient at least twice a year for 5-8 days at a time or in the Emergency Room at least 3-4 times a year? That is how I lived my life as if I had no choice to have a better life, just a sickly life.

In 2001, I started working with a medical insurance company as a Customer Service Representative. As I was receiving calls, I heard similar stories to my own. This is when I began to ask myself why. Although I had asked myself these questions in the past, I didn't know enough at the time to answer the question; however, as I got older and had a family to look after, I started to conduct my own research. I also started to research the many aliments and chronic conditions that I heard on the phone calls from the policyholders.

Years later I got a promotion at the insurance company working alongside nurses and doctors. It was their job to review certain cases and determine what was medical necessary. I would have conversations with the nurses about all types of chronic illnesses, including asthma. (Mind you, I would sometimes take nebulizer treatments at work.) The nurses let me know that not only did my allergies contribute to my asthma attacks, but also my diet! Although I cooked and took my breakfast and lunch, it was not always healthy. I would come home on a Wednesday evening, cook collard greens with smoked turkey necks or neckbones, baked macaroni and cheese, corn bread, fried chicken and ham and wouldn't think twice about what I was putting into my body. In my mind, it couldn't be all that bad. Man, homemade fried chicken was and still is my weakness! I could eat it every single day if I could, but after my conversations with the nurses I learned it is not very healthy.

Unfortunately, all that cooking and good eating caught up to me. In 2007, I was diagnosed with diabetes. My doctor informed me that I needed to lose weight, exercise and eat better. I immediately thought to myself, "Oh no, no more fried chicken!" I was thinking about the food I had to give UP, not about changing my lifestyle. When I went to work the next day, I spoke with one of the nurses again and let her know my latest illness. I told her that if I did not get it together my doctor said that I may have to be on insulin. The thought of giving myself a needle scared the living daylights out of me. The nurse asked me if I wanted her help and if so, she was willing to help. However, for her to help me, she had certain conditions. I would have to be willing to listen to what she's telling me, and to work on giving up a few of my bad habits. I told her yes, I am ready to make the necessary changes for the betterment of my life. Lord knows I had no idea what I was saying yes to when I asked for help! I was a person who cooked daily. When I went to work, I took what I cooked for dinner the night before. Most times, what I brought to work was unhealthy, so she took the time to educate me on what I was eating and explained why it was unhealthy. She would make sure I understood that it was about how the food was prepared AND the TYPE of food. I remember her throwing my food in the trash and taking me to the restaurant to grab a healthy meal. It was that very moment that I decided to begin my Health and Wellness journey.

I soon joined Bally's gym. I started exercising 7 days a week. Even if all I could do was walk or ride on the bike, I made sure I did something. I was determined to find a way to get off those medications (I was taking Actos and Metformin and boy were they nasty!), and stop pricking my finger 3 times a day. I hated it! There were 90 days in between my next doctor's appointment so I had to get on the ball. I gave myself 90 days of being disciplined, focused and determined to become knowledgeable about the true meaning of healthy eating. When I went back to the doctor's, I had lost some weight however, my sugar level was still high. It took a little over a year to really get the full understanding of where I needed to be with my numbers as well as how I desired to live my life. All I knew was that I wanted to live.

Over the next several years, my goals were to learn the true meaning of living a healthy lifestyle. Due to my diligence, not only did I come off my medications for diabetes, it also lessened my asthma attacks. Also, around this time, I started to attend church on a regular basis. I began to pray more about the life that I wanted to lead and live. This part of my journey was not only for myself but for my children as well. I needed my children to know that I was serious about living a healthy lifestyle. As I began to get more into the word, I learned about the Fruits of the Spirit. I realized that I needed to grow personally in all 9 fruits if I truly wanted to live a fulfilled life without regrets.

The strength of the Lord carried me during this time, through my good days and my bad days. However, in 2017, I was dealt another blow; I was diagnosed with Fibromyalgia. It is a diagnosis that has become more common in America. In fact, Fibromyalgia "Affects 3.7 million people between the ages of 40-75. It is a disease that is a constellation of systems that can be managed. However, there are several triggers such as physical trauma, emotional trauma or hormonal changes may trigger the development of generalized pain, fatigue and sleep disturbances that cause symptoms."(Arthritis.org) While researching, learning, and experimenting, I came to the realization that my triggers include physical exertion, and stress. I wasn't complaining about

9

the pain or discomfort I was experiencing, nor was I talking about it to anyone because I attributed it to working out too much. I never realized the pain was an actual illness.

Here is where the Fruits of the Spirt I told you about earlier helped me. They helped me to created five things I do daily:

1. I determined what my daily activities would be and write them down.
   a. I wanted to be healthier by eating healthier foods.
   b. I wanted to love more, therefore, I started practicing being kind to others and learning how to love everyone despite their own challenges.
   c. I needed peace in my life. I started creating ways to be peaceful, so I started meditating.
   d. My physical abilities were limited but I still wanted to move so I started practicing Yoga more.
   e. I needed to be more focused, so I started learning more about essential oils and their properties.
2. My life was a little chaotic at this time because I was trying to do too many things at once while being all things to all people - thus excluding myself. I had to prioritize my goals, my life and I had to learn how to pray. Here are few affirmations I would say to myself:
   a. I am less stressed.
   b. I have a sweet and caring spirit.
   c. I can maintain a more positive attitude.
   d. I am more focused on daily tasks.
   e. I accomplish more in a day.
3. You cannot make decisions based off of your feelings; when you make emotional decisions, you often regret the decision you just made. Here are a few ideas to help you:
   a. Know what you need. If you need a book, get it.
   b. If you need to listen to positive thinking daily, do it.

c. Don't have time to read but love learning, start listening to audio books.

d. Having trouble getting started? Start out with just 10 minutes a day, reading, exercising, walking etc. More importantly, just start even if it is small.

4. You can't do the same things each year and expect a change. In order to live and be happy, you must fight for it. Hebrews 12:11 states, "No discipline is enjoyable while it is happening, it's painful! But afterward, there will be a peaceful harvest of right living for those who are trained in this way." Here are a few things to look forward to through hard work and discipline:

   a. A life that is full of abundance and happiness.
   b. To sustain peace in my life regardless of my illness.
   c. To make a difference by helping others understand their worth.
   d. To be pain-free.
   e. To be grateful every single day of my life.

5. After taking time to write down our goals and how we want to live, you must evaluate your process to determine your progress. Here are a few questions to ask yourself:

   a. How am I doing as far as eating healthy?
   b. How am I overcoming my challenges?
   c. Have I created peace within my life? If not, what changes do I need to make?
   d. Have I been focusing on my goals and making positive changes? If not, why?

COACHING ASSIGNMENT

Above, I offered you some recommendations that have helped me through my journey for wellness, good health, and peace. As you consider my journey, I would like for you to consider your own journey by:

- Creating 5 daily activities that you would like to accomplish.
- Prioritize your goals.
- Create ideas regarding how you can enjoy what you are trying to accomplish.
- Know your "why."
- Evaluate your process and progress.

Here is the fun part! Now that you have thought about it, I want to encourage you to take 30 minutes for the activities below:

Name 5 activities that you wish to accomplish daily:

1. _____

2. _____

3. _____

4. _____

5. _____

Now, prioritize the 5 goals that you have created:

1. _____

2. _____

   _____
3. _____

   _____
4. _____

   _____
5. _____

   _____

Create 5 ways you can enjoy accomplishing your goals:
1. _____

   _____
2. _____

   _____
3. _____

   _____
4. _____

   _____
5. _____

   _____

Create the top 5 things that define your "why":
1. _____

   _____
2. _____

   _____
3. _____

   _____
4. _____

   _____
5. _____

   _____

Write down 5 ways you will evaluate your process and progress:

1. _____
   _____
2. _____
   _____
3. _____
   _____
4. _____
   _____
5. _____
   _____

Now that you have written your 5 Daily Living Attributes, go to the Lord in prayer to seek guidance, clarity, strength, and support through your personal journey. Being as though this is a guided book; I am offering you the prayer that has kept me. You can always create one for yourself, but since I am not a coach who will leave you out there alone, I wanted to give you an option. Is that alright? It might be a bit cliché, but I love the Serenity prayer:

God grant me the serenity to accept the things I cannot change; Courage to change the things I can; And wisdom to know the difference.

Living one day at a time; Enjoying one moment at a time; Accepting hardships as the pathway to peace; Taking, as He did, this sinful world As it is, not as I would have it; Trusting that He will make all things right If I surrender to His Will; So that I may be reasonably happy in this life And supremely happy with Him Forever and ever in the next. Amen. (prayer attributed to Reinhold Neibuhr, 1892-1971)

https://www.lords-prayer-words.com/famous_prayers/god_grant_me_the_serenity.html

Mind

C ~ COMPASSION

When you turn on the news, there are often stories about killings, accidents, and politics that are delivered in a negative light. When you open your social media, there are a ton of messages of someone passing away, someone losing their home or plan old fashioned bullying. Oftentimes it is hard to stay positive when there seems to be so much negativity in the world. With so many things happening, having negative self-talk is easy and can feel normal. This is when compassion is needed. Below are a few things to consider:

How can you feel complete when you can't think straight?

How can you feel compassion when everything around you is going wrong?

How can you love yourself or others when the images in your head are about death, hurt, ignorance, hatred, and evil?

How can you move on when you have been hurt by a loved one, disrespected, lose your home or feel like you have lost your independence?

I believe that we as people are capable of compassion, however with all that is going on its hard for us to express it. We must do our best to guard our minds by continuously working on our individual, spiritual, and emotional well-being.

When was the last time you took an audit of your life? I started to take inventory of the type of deposits I was putting in my mind. I absolutely love watching the Cooking Channel because I find it positive. I find that when I allowed positivity to enter my subconscious, it allows my compassion to come forth. Even if you listen to gospel, or watch something positive on YouTube, or just sit down and read a self-help book, can help contribute to your mental and emotional wellness, which ultimately helps you to realize your compassion.

One of the first things I started working on for myself is having more compassion. Compassion for others is very important, however, SELF-compassion is equally important. At this point of my life I had no idea what self-compassion truly meant until I researched it. I started to reading blogs and articles that focused on self-compassion to get a better understanding of how to accomplish this. Here's what I found:

Compassion is the ability to understand a person's feelings. Self-compassion is the ability to understand your OWN feelings. This may sound simple, but for me at least it was a concept that took me a while to grasp. I asked myself why this is so hard for me to do. To help me find an answer, I joined several women's groups; and we all shared our stories. I noticed that for women (especially mothers) it's difficult because we are nurturers and are often to put others before ourselves.

Below are a few tips to help with your self-compassion:

- **Be okay with being imperfect.** There is no such thing as perfection. Too often women are hard on themselves because of the way they look, feel, walk, talk or act and the reality is we can all use some sort of improvement.
- **Be kind to yourself.** Ask yourself, have you been kind to yourself lately? If so, how were you kind to yourself? (Write it down in your journal). Take a good look at what you have

19

accomplished over the previous week and be brutally honest.

- **Practice Forgiveness.** Most of us have things that we would like to change from our past, but the reality is, all we can do is accept whatever has happened, learn from it, forgive ourselves and others and move forward.
- **Be Mindful and Live in the moment.** Wait, what does that even mean? It means to be grateful for the moment that God has allowed you to experience! I know this can difficult to do, but it is very necessary for your emotional and mental wellness. In addition, you can use different apps that can help you live in the moment. I like using an App called "Calm" (Meditate, Sleep, Relax). It is a leading app for anxiety, stress, and so much more. I highly recommend this app, and the great thing about it is that it's free (however, the more advanced options require a fee).
- **Express gratitude.** Take 1 minute and look at your surroundings and ask yourself these questions. (Write it down in your journal):
  - Did you wake up this morning?
  - What did you have for breakfast?
  - Were you able to take a shower and brush your teeth?
  - Do you have a home to come back to once you leave the house?

If you answered these questions positively, then you should be grateful. Most blessings come in the form of having a roof over your head, clothes on your back, and food on the table. We should show gratitude for these little things.

According to Colossians 3:12; "Therefore, as God's chosen people, holy and dearly loved, clothe yourselves with compassion, kindness, humility, gentleness, and patience."

Now it's your turn. I would like for you to take 10 minutes and think about what you need to work on for yourself. You can choose any word that starts with the letter C (ex. Calm, Celebrate, Collaborate, Comfort to name a few).

COACHING ASSIGNMENT

1. What word did you choose for the letter C?

    _____

    _____

    _____

    _____

2. What is the definition or bible verses for your word?

    _____

    _____

    _____

    _____

3. Why did you choose this word?

    _____

    _____

    _____

    _____

4. How did you feel when you started thinking about your word?

    _____

    _____

    _____

    _____

5. How can you incorporate your word into your daily lifestyle?

    _____

    _____

_____

_____

Now, I want to encourage you to take 15-30 minutes and create your own list.

Name 5 things that you feel you that you can improve on:

1. _____
   _____

2. _____
   _____

3. _____
   _____

4. _____
   _____

5. _____
   _____

Going by the list of the things that you can improve on, turn them into a positive affirmations:

1. _____
   _____

2. _____
   _____

3. _____
   _____

4. _____
   _____

5. _____
   _____

Create 5 ways you will be kind to yourself:

1. _____
   _____

2. _____

3. _____

4. _____

5. _____

Create the 5 ways you are going to be more mindful and live in the moment:

1. _____

2. _____

3. _____

4. _____

5. _____

Write down 5 things you are grateful for:

1. _____

2. _____

3. _____

4. _____

5. _____

O ~ OVERLOOKED

I chose the word Overlooked because that is exactly what happened to me as a child (especially due to my illnesses), however, even more so as an adult. Having an ailment causes people treat you differently; they don't mean to, but the fact remains the same. As a child it was hard for me to understand why, and I could not put into words the way it made me feel. As an adult I have a better understanding of why, and I can sum it up all into one phrase: being overlooked.

I have been a chronic asthmatic pretty much my entire life, which means that I can't run for a long distance, but the one thing I can do is run sprints! Many of our games growing up consisted of lots of running, such as dodge ball, tag and racing. Although I played these games, I had to take a lot of breaks. After a while, your friends would stop asking you play these games because kids for the most part do not show compassion – which ultimately leads to being overlooked. Who could blame them? Who wants to take breaks when playing tag?

As an adult, things really didn't get any easier. I was being overlooked job opportunities in my professional life as well as having very few meaningful friendships in my personal life. Although I have always considered myself a great employee, I also missed a lot of work due to my illnesses. When you think about someone who is a good employee, you think about someone who is loyal, dependable, selfless, attentive and goal oriented. Unfortunately, the best ability is availability. Availability = appreciation; being unavailable = being overlooked.

I was introduced by a good friend of mine to something that has helped me even to this day: Personal Development. "What in the heck does Personal Development mean?" I asked my friend. She started out by asking ME questions; about my life, my work, church, etc. She introduced me to Jim Rohn, Les Brown, and Warren Buffet. I quickly realized that I allowed other people's perception of me – such as being overlooked – define who I am. As I started reading the Personal Development books by those individuals, I saw that at one point or another they were overlooked too, however they stopped allowing other people to define who they were as a certain point.

I continued with my Personal Development by attending classes in areas that I identified that I needed to grow. I would attend different conferences all to help me grow and become successful yet realized that although it helped, it didn't transform me because I was not applying anything I learned. I was subconsciously still allowing myself to be defined by other people. I was just someone learning and not growing, and I knew that I had to change my mindset if I didn't want to continue to be overlooked.

When you are being overlooked for a job, by your significant other, a friend and other people in your life, just know that you are right where God wants you to be. Understand that you may feel as if you are being overlooked because you care too much about what other people think of you. This needs to change because until you have faith in your own abilities, you will always feel as if you are being overlooked.

- Start focusing on the small victories and write them down in your journal at the end of each week.

- Created goals based on what you need to accomplish each day and make them small. By doing so, you will not feel overwhelmed or disappointed if it doesn't get completed.
- Instead of thinking you can handle everything by yourself (the reality is we all need help), reach out to others for guidance.
- Personal Development is a process and can take months and even years to develop but you must be patient with yourself.

COACHING ASSIGNMENT

Can you think about how you feel when you are overwhelmed or feel overlooked? Come up with some of your own ideas on how you can help yourself?

Name 5 things that makes you feel like you are being overlooked:

1. _____
_____
2. _____
_____
3. _____
_____
4. _____
_____
5. _____
_____

Now, write why do you feel you are being overlooked: You cannot grow without finding out why you feel that way.

1. _____
_____
2. _____
_____
3. _____
_____
4. _____
_____
5. _____
_____

Write 5 things you will do for yourself to overcome the feeling of being overlooked:

1. _____
   _____
2. _____
   _____
3. _____
   _____
4. _____
   _____
5. _____
   _____

Create the 5 ways you can stay motivated when you are feeling unappreciated:

1. _____
   _____
2. _____
   _____
3. _____
   _____
4. _____
   _____
5. _____
   _____

Write down 5 things you are grateful for in this subject:

1. _____
   _____
2. _____
   _____

3. _____

_____

4. _____

_____

5. _____

_____

M ~ MINDSET

Anything you do in life starts with your mindset. Just as we discussed being overlooked in the previous chapter, changing your mindset will help you overcome it. When I was a child, I would see my parents fussing, yelling, and cussing at each other and I thought that was how adults communicated. Before I met my husband, I thought I was the world's greatest communicator; that was my mindset at that time. When we would have disagreements, I would yell, cuss and fight because that is what I was used to. He would stop me in the middle of me acting a fool and explain that adults communicate effectively by calmly discussing the issue to get your point across. What he was doing (without stated it) was changing my mindset. This was a totally different way I was used to, and it took some time. The thing is, I didn't realize how bad it was for me UNTIL I was able to make that mindset shift.

It has also helped me in other areas of my life, even in writing this book. It wasn't an easy transition, but it has paid off. Mindset means "a mental attitude, inclination or a fixed state of mind." (Webster's Dictionary). Change is inevitable but oftentimes it is hard to embrace the change. Think about how many times your doctor has told you that you need to either lose weight or gain weight. What about that friend that you talk to about your problems, and the feedback you get from them is negative? There is almost nothing that hinders mindset shifts more than to get negative feedback, especially from someone who you respect.

In order to embrace change, it starts with our thoughts. We decide how we act or react to situations. It's important to be intentional about our life because only YOU can live it. This sounds like a great plan, but sometimes it's the last thing on our list of priorities. We focus more on our jobs, our families, our businesses, our relationships, but not ourselves. Taking control over your mindset takes time, diligence and practice. In fact, it can take months or even years before you see any positive results. Also, you must understand that setbacks will happen.

Below is a list of things that you can do that can help you start to change your mindset:

1. Started speaking life into yourself.
2. Focus on the positive things you have accomplished each day.
3. Have a clear vision of how you want your life to look and feel.
4. Build your belief system and know that you are worth it.
5. Find a coach or mentor who can help you overcome your obstacles.

Here are some more things you can do to help you:

Affirmations
- I am extremely excited that I have more money than I need to live and be happy.
- I am living in my truth.
- I am responsible for who I am, not others and do not need their validation.
- I am so happy and grateful for my job, family and business.
- I am ecstatic that I am the healthiest I have ever been.

I know that this can be a bit cliché and you've heard this before, but affirmations do work. Along with the affirmations I had to also become a master of how I feel and change my mood when necessary, especially when someone has upset me. When I feel like my world is closing in on me and I am about to explode, there are a few things that I do to aid in changing my mood.

- I think about the situation and breathe for 10 seconds before I respond.
- If I don't have to respond quickly, I take a break and listen to Tye Tribbett. My mood changes as soon as the music comes on.
- If I'm unable to do either of the two and at a computer, I type out my feelings to get what I am feeling off my chest, so I won't regret responding.
- If it's something that I can wait to respond, sometimes I will wait 24 hours before responding.
- Lastly, I sing to myself.

Oftentimes, I see the situation for what it is and acknowledge it, which is also part of your mindset change. I have learned that it's not always me to create my feelings, but I learned to count all my blessing even down to the smallest details. Our actions speak louder than our words and getting control of our actions are very important for our sanity. Below is a list of things I have learned:

- I have learned the importance of thinking before I react to a situation.
- I have learned that I must be childlike and listen.
- I had to learn to stop comparing myself to others because that did not help either.

- I had to learn how to be unbiased. Thus, separating how I was feeling from what was being discussed. My husband would always say, start seeing things for what they are and not what I wanted them to be.

As I previously stated, I had to overcome how I saw food. This was also a mindset shift. You could have never told me that I was an emotional eater. When I think of emotional eating, I think of eating for every sadness or eating everything in sight. In my mind, I wasn't eating every time I felt hungry, upset or angry. I was conscious about eating 5/6 small meals a day, but when something happened that I had no control over, I would eat unhealthy foods. My husband made me realize that although I was not overeating, it was still considered emotional eating. I had to learn and am still learning that my body is God's temple and we have control over how we live our lives. Below are a few things that I started to do for myself:

- I started to eat mindfully.
- I eat when I get hungry and journal my feelings each time I eat or drink anything to determine my intentions.
- I eat for nourishment instead of just eating.
- I eat until I am satisfied.
- I don't always get this part right because of the family but I try to remove the foods that will go against my goals.

The key is learning to take control over how you think, feel and react to situations that may not be the easiest to handle it. No, you won't get it right all the time. However, when you create a process it will help you to overcome any obstacle that comes your way. This will help you to be better prepared to deal with the situation at hand. I want you to think about the last time you got angry because of what someone said or did to you. Write down:

- What were you thinking?
- How did it make you feel?
- How did you respond?
- Was it in a positive or negative way?
- What could you have done differently based on how you answered your above questions?

COACHING ASSIGNMENT

Name 5 things you can do to overcome how you are feeling in the moment:

1. _____

2. _____

3. _____

4. _____

5. _____

Now, write down 5 positive ways on how you can respond to those feelings.

1. _____

2. _____

3. _____

4. _____

5. _____

Write 5 affirmations that will help with changing your mindset:

1. _____
   _____

2. _____
   _____

3. _____
   _____

4. _____
   _____

5. _____
   _____

Create 5 positive things you will do before reacting to a situation that is good, bad or indifferent:

1. _____
   _____

2. _____
   _____

3. _____
   _____

4. _____
   _____

5. _____
   _____

Write down 5 ways you have a positive relationship with food:

1. _____
   _____

2. _____
   _____

3. _____
   _____

4. _____

_____

5. _____

_____

P~PROGRESS, NOT PERFECTION

So far, we discussed how important it is to have compassion, how you can overcome the feeling of being overlooked, and about changing our mindsets. It is not fair to expect major changes for things that you have been dealing with for many years; believe it or not this is also part of the process. It's going to take time. You must allow all the time you need to overcome your obstacles. It's going to take more than a 30-day challenge or just completing the assignments in this book. It's going to take daily action, prayer, journaling, being honest about your feelings and seeking help from a professional if necessary. Trauma is no joke and if you have unresolved trauma, it's going to make it more difficult to overcome your obstacles because you cannot mask everything. That's why it's important to understand that all progress is a process and there is no such thing as perfection, we all have areas where we can grow.

When I speak with other women, the one thing I hear the most is "I want to look and feel amazing when I look in the mirror..." Then I ask, "Why don't you feel amazing now?" More often or not women are dissatisfied with their physical appearance. I know the feeling!

As I continue to make improvements in my life, I am learning that it's not just about the accomplishments you achieved

44

but how you celebrate them. Personal Development has taught me that it is not about materialistic things that made me feel better, it was understanding that no one is perfect and there will always be room for growth. I am here to tell you that progress is not perfection, it is also understanding that ALL process is progress, even when the results are hard to see. Celebrate the little things. While this is still a struggle for me, there are a few things that I have been doing that has helped me in this process. Below are a few recommendations that you can do to help you:

Strive for Daily Improvement

This part of the process does work, even if it doesn't seem like you're making the improvements. Also, this part of the process can be frustrating, but try to persevere. A friend of mine (Nicole) runs a class where she teaches how to "Mind Map." Mind Mapping is a technique that focuses on breaking down your goals every three months or so. This helps you move from "brainstorming" to "strategizing", along with creating an action plan of attainable tasks. I took this class because I needed help to become more organized. After learning this technique and applying it, I was able to clearly define my goals for my personal and professional life. Through this process, I have learned that every coach needs a coach. I had to allow myself to be coached and do the work required for me to learn and grow, which is a very important part of my process.

Below are a few things that I do daily to strive for improvement:

- Create an intention for the day.
- Write down 1 goal that I need to accomplish.
- Write down my accomplishments in my journal.
- Show gratitude for the goal that was completed, even if you only completed part of it.

Be Consistent

Understanding that being consistent is also part of the process. Creating daily habits is a great way to develop consistency, as long as you are honest and stay focused and on task at hand.

Below are a few things that I do daily to create consistency in my life:

- Pray
- Read my daily devotion
- Read my personal development for business
- Stretch, Plank and most days exercise.
- 1 hour a day I work my business goals

Remember Why started

Consistency is the most important part of the process! Without consistency, the process breaks down. I recently had a conversation with my daughter (who is nineteen). She has been doing hair for several years now, however she is frustrated because she is not where she wants to be in her career. I often remind her to remember all she has accomplished at her age and to constantly ask herself, why she's doing what she's doing. After she has taken time to remember why she started doing hair, it clicks. She is now able to strive for success and be consistent. In turn it will eventually, pay off.

COACHING ASSIGNMENT

Name 5 things you can daily to show improvements on your goals:

1. _____
   _____
2. _____
   _____
3. _____
   _____
4. _____
   _____
5. _____
   _____

Now, write down 5 positive ways you can stay consistent:

1. _____
   _____
2. _____
   _____
3. _____
   _____
4. _____
   _____
5. _____
   _____

Write down your Why and why you got started:

_____
_____
_____

Body

L ~ LIFE'S VISION

Let's talk about lifestyle and Life's Vision. We have talked about having self-compassion, being overlooked, working on our mindsets, along with progress and process. Your Life's Vision is where you see yourself 5, 10, or 15 years from now and the journey and process it takes for you to get there. Everybody's Life's Vision is different, and they also may change based on the circumstances that happen in your life. When you think about each of the topics in the previous chapters, each of these are in some way connected to our lifestyle.

We are all in control over our lifestyles and if we are not living our best life it's usually because of the decisions we have made in our lives. When you focus on the things that you can control and worry about less about the things that are beyond your control, you will start to see a change in your mindset which leads to a change in your lifestyle. Once you see the change in your lifestyle, then your Life's Vision comes more into focus.

What have you envisioned for your life? Do you want a large home, with a fence and a huge backyard? Are you looking to be financially independent? Do you want to live your best life as healthy as you can be? I used to want to be rich, have a large home where I can have parties and feel free. However, after becoming an entrepreneur, and working toward my goals, I learned that being rich didn't necessarily equate to happiness.

Have you taken the time to identify your Life's Vision? It's something we should revisit often, and I want you to take this time to think what you want for your life in the next year? Where do you see yourself in a year? What steps are you going to take get you to your next goal? Are you being realistic about your goals? When was the last time you revisited your vision board?

Take some time and think about your Life's Vision. Be very specific. You may have to break down each goal and its action steps down to the smallest detail. Having a poster board filled with pictures of your milestones, family members, future aspirations (also called a vision board), can help you to see your vision clearly every time you look at it.

E ~ EARLY DETECTION

According to the American Medical Association (AMA), early detection refers to measures that can be taken to diagnosis cancer as early as possible; this is crucial to cancer treatment because the earliest that it's detected the easier it is to treat. As it pertains to Health and Wellness, and all of the topics we have covered so far, early detection refers to preventive care; meaning that you know your body well enough to realize something is wrong even if you don't know what that something is.

Early detection as it pertains to Health and Wellness is about being aware of our mental, emotional, and physical well-being, and *noticing any adverse changes*. This means that you absolutely have to know your mental, emotional and physical levels.

Normal mental health diagnoses – such as depression, anxiety, bipolarism, ect. – are typically given by a licensed mental doctor. However, mental early detection pertains to paying attention to YOUR current mental health level and noticing any changes. This can be difficult because these changes can be hard to detect. The best prevention is to seek professional help if you do notice a change.

Emotional early detection is the same as mental early detection; indeed, these two go hand in hand. Also, as with mental health, early detection starts with your current emotional state. The problem with this is that your emotions can change in an instant. If you do notice any major changes in your emotions from one minute to the next, you can seek professional help. However, this can also be accomplished by hiring a coach, getting a few self-help books and writing in a journal.

Physical early detection is a lot more straight-forward than either mental or emotional early detection. This consists of regular visits to your primary care doctor, exercise, healthy eating and just simply paying attention to your body.

Below is a list of recommendations for basic physical early detections (obtained from https://www.cdc.gov/cancer/breast/basic_info/mammograms.htm):

Here are a few tips for getting a Mammogram:
- Try not to have your mammogram the week before you get your period our during your period because your beast maybe tender or swollen.
- During your appointment, you are not allowed to wear deodorant, perfume or powder because they will show up as white dots on the X-Ray.
- Don't be so afraid of the results that you make excuses on why you can't get an appointment.

Here are some basic recommendations based on the Affordable Care Act (https://www.healthcare.gov/preventive-care-adults/):

- Abdominal aortic aneurysm one-time screening for men of specified ages who have ever smoked
- Alcohol misuse screening and counseling
- Aspirin use to prevent cardiovascular disease and colorectal cancer for adults 50 to 59 years with a high cardiovascular risk
- Blood pressure screening
- Cholesterol screening for adults of certain ages or at higher risk
- Colorectal cancer screening for adults 50 to 75
- Depression screening
- Diabetes (Type 2) screening for adults 40 to 70 years who are overweight or obese
- Diet counseling for adults at higher risk for chronic disease
- Falls prevention (with exercise or physical therapy and vitamin D use) for adults 65 years and over, living in a community setting
- Hepatitis B screening ⬈ for people at high risk, including people from countries with 2% or more Hepatitis B prevalence, and U.S.-born people not vaccinated as infants and with at least one parent born in a region with 8% or more Hepatitis B prevalence.
- Hepatitis C screening for adults at increased risk, and one time for everyone born 1945–1965
- HIV screening for everyone ages 15 to 65, and other ages at increased risk
- Immunization vaccines for adults — doses, recommended ages, and recommended populations vary:
  - Diphtheria
  - Hepatitis A
  - Hepatitis B
  - Herpes Zoster
  - Human Papillomavirus (HPV)

- o Influenza (flu shot)
- o Measles
- o Meningococcal
- o Mumps
- o Pertussis
- o Pneumococcal
- o Tetanus
- o Varicella (Chickenpox)
- Lung cancer screening for adults 55-80 at high risk for lung cancer because they're heavy smokers or have quit in the past 15 years
- Obesity screening and counseling
- Sexually transmitted infection (STI) prevention counseling for adults at higher risk
- Statin preventive medication for adults 40 to 75 at high risk
- Syphilis screening for adults at higher risk
- Tobacco use screening for all adults and cessation interventions for tobacco users
- Tuberculosis screening for certain adults without symptoms at high risk

Ladies, I want you to take some time and think about the last time you had Obstetrician Gynecologist (OBGYN) appointment or a Primary care Physician (PCP) appointment. Think about some things that have been happening to your body, write them down and have them ready for your next appointment

Doctor's Name	Telephone Number	Appointment Date	What have I been experiencing lately?

Now that you have made your appointments, it's time to make changes based on the results provided by the doctor.

T ~ TIME OUT

A typical day in our lives usually consist of creating a daily routine. Many of us work a job that requires 9 to 10 hours of our time a day. If you don't live close to your job, it will require you to commute to and from work and that can take an additional hour or two of your time. If you are a parent and have children in school, you have to give them time to help with homework and cook dinner, which takes up more of your time. If you are married or have a significant other, you have to spend time with them as well. Now, you have went through your entire day and none of this consisted of you doing anything for yourself!

Now it's the weekend and you are exhausted; you are thinking about all the things that you have to do for everyone else and are feeling overwhelmed. You are overwhelmed because you have not taken any Time Out for yourself because you have given all your time to everyone, your job, your husband, your friends and family. A good friend of mine told me that I have to take time for myself because there will always be more work to do. There are only 24 hours in a day, and we deserve at least 1 hour for ourselves daily.

Taking Time Out for yourself can also help you with your emotional and physical health because you will take to deal with your emotions, exercise or eat healthier. Over exertion can cause more problems because stress if the number 1 killer, which is why we MUST all have a Time Out. It is very imperative that we all take a break and enjoy some fresh air or even get away for a weekend.

Below are a few ideas that you can use to take a Time Out:

- You can start taking classes for Yoga. This can help to reduce your anxiety and aid in getting some rest.
- You can create a routine to pray at night before bed to help ease your mind from your busy day.
- Meditation can teach you how to rid the noise you hear in your head because you are thinking about everything you haven't accomplished for the day.
- If you are a coffee drinker, limit the amount of caffeine you are drinking throughout the day.
- Changing your diet can also help with taking time out because you are focusing on better health.
- Using essential oils is another way to help you with Time Out. The oils all have their own properties on how they can assist you with meditation, breathing, resting and pure relaxation.
- Taking some time to work directly with a therapist can also help you take Time Out for yourself because you are focusing on different areas of your life with them.
- My last recommendation is a book called "Rest Well"; God's gift for a good night's sleep written by Stacey Speller. It's an amazing book that you can get that can also help you take a Time Out. In this book, the main point that resonated with me was the scripture in Psalms 127:2, "It's useless to rise early and go to bed late and work your worried fingers to

the bone. Don't you know he enjoys giving rest to those He love". Man, this was powerful, and the rest of her book helped me so much I had to give her a shout out.

Take a few minutes to brain dump and write down everything that comes to mind. You will be surprised of the things you never left go that you thought you did!

_____
_____
_____
_____
_____
_____
_____
_____
_____
_____
_____
_____
_____
_____
_____
_____

I ~ INSURANCE (HEALTH & LIFE)

Health Insurance

I have been working in the medical insurance industry for over Twenty years and it never ceases to amaze me how many of us do not understand how medical coverage works. In a chapter that dealt with early detection, I talked about why it's important to make our doctor's appointment and different types of preventive care. In this section we are going to talk about why it's important to have medical coverage.

Before I started working at a medical insurance company, I had no clue about medical insurance or its importance. While working at the company, I learned about how coverages worked, premiums, and the importance of seeing your doctor. I was amazed at what I was seeing when the medical bills were coming in and they are over $80,000 for a 5 day stay in the hospital. Most importantly, I learned how having medical coverage saved money, as well as saved lives. The fact is that people who have coverage used it, however, people that didn't have coverage did not seek care when they needed it.

Did you know that some doctors don't not always accept your medical insurance? There is a different language in the medical insurance world and unless someone educates you, you are clueless.

What does an IN-Network (INN) provider mean? It means that the doctor you have chosen to see has a contract with the health plan and regardless of how much they charge, they will accept to be paid a certain amount.

What does an Out-of-network (OON) provider mean? It means that the doctor you have chosen to see does not contract with your health plan and regardless of what the health plan will pay, ultimately, you are responsible to the total amount billed. Typically, when you see an OON provider you are paying them upfront and sending in a request for reimbursement from your health plan.

I could write a whole book on this, but I just want to give a few highlights on why you should do all you can to ensure you have medical coverage regardless of where you are getting from. You can get it through the Marketplace, your Employer, Medicare, or Medical Assistance, which is through the state.

1. Most of us cannot afford one trip to the emergency so we don't go, which makes matters worse.
2. Most of us cannot afford the medication. My one medication called Symbicort is $500 before applied to my medical insurance. I cannot afford this one mediation without it and I have six different medications. Imagine if I didn't have medical coverage, I would have to go without my medication, which has helped keep me from having a major issue.

3. We make excuses on why we cannot afford to get medical coverage. While this is the case for many people, somethings should be non-negotiable because it can save your life in the long run.
4. You are less worried when you must make a trip to the doctor or have a medical condition that requires many trips to the doctor.
5. When you are ill, your family can help you seek care without thinking about how they are going to pay for this visit. Now, there are some situations that you will feel this way, but when you are covered for the larger portions, you can worry about your responsibilities later.

Life Insurance

Having life insurance is just as important as having medical coverage. You have three options when selecting a life insurance policy: you can either purchase one through your job, financial institution, or through a private company. While getting a life insurance policy through your employer may seem like the most convenient option, it's not without its drawbacks. If you were to lose your job, you would lose your life insurance coverage (which is also known as *term life coverage*). You could also have a lapse in coverage if you were to quit your job and find a new job. Another thing to consider is whether your company's standard life insurance policy is large enough if you have a spouse and other dependents. If not, you may have to purchase a supplemental policy from an outside entity. If at all possible, try to get whole life coverage. (see chart below)

Before we move into the types of policies there are, let me explain what a life insurance policy is. A life insurance policy is a contract with an insurance company, in which the insurance company provides a lump-sum payment (also known as a death benefits) to beneficiaries upon the insured's death. Typically, life insurance is chosen based on the needs and goals of the policy owner. Term life insurance generally provides protection for a set period, while permanent insurance – such as whole and universal life – provides lifetime coverage. It's important to note that death benefits from all types of life insurance are generally income tax free.

Term life insurance

Term life insurance is designed to provide financial protection for a specific period, such as 10 or 20 years. With traditional term insurance, the premium payment amount stays the same for the coverage period you select. After that period, policies may offer continued coverage, usually at a substantially higher premium payment rate.

In addition, term life insurance proceeds can be used to replace lost potential income during working years. This can provide a safety net for your beneficiaries and can also help ensure the family's financial goals will still be met—goals like paying off a mortgage, keeping a business running, and paying for college. It's important to note that, although term life can be used to replace lost potential income, life insurance benefits are paid at one time in a lump sum, not in regular payments like paychecks.

Universal life insurance

Universal life insurance is a type of permanent life insurance designed to provide lifetime coverage. Unlike whole life insurance, universal life insurance policies are flexible and may allow you to raise or lower your premium payment or coverage amounts throughout your lifetime. Universal life insurance is most often used as part of a flexible estate planning strategy to help preserve wealth to be transferred to beneficiaries. Another common use is long term income replacement, where the need extends beyond working years. Some universal life insurance product designs focus on providing both death benefit coverage and building cash value while others focus on providing guaranteed death benefit coverage.

Whole life insurance

Whole life insurance is a type of permanent life insurance designed to provide lifetime coverage. Because of the lifetime coverage period, whole life usually has higher premium payments than term life. Policy premium payments are typically fixed, and, unlike term, whole life has a cash value, which functions as a savings component and may accumulate tax-deferred over time. Whole life can be used as an estate planning tool to help preserve the wealth you plan to transfer to your beneficiaries.

The chart below is a comparison between the different types of life insurance:

Comparing Types of Life Insurance			
	Term Life Insurance	**Universal Life Insurance**	**Whole Life Insurance**
Needs it helps meet	Income replacement during working years	Wealth transfer, income protection and some designs focus on tax-deferred wealth accumulation	Wealth transfer, preservation and, tax-deferred wealth accumulation
Protection period	Designed for a specific period (usually several years)	Flexible; generally, for a lifetime	For a lifetime
Cost differences	Typically, less expensive than permanent	Generally, more expensive than term	Generally, more expensive than term
Premiums	Typically fixed	Flexible	Typically fixed
Proceeds paid to beneficiaries	Yes, generally income tax-free	Yes, generally income tax-free	Yes, generally income tax-free
Investment options	No	No[2]	No
May help build equity	No	Yes	Yes

O~ OWN YOUR TRUTH (Tranquility)

Own your Truth

Owning your truth means being open, honest and authentic to yourself. I have conversations with my 19-year-old daughter about this, and the one thing that bugs her the most is when people are not being their authentic selves or doing things to please other people. If you look at your social media, you can honestly say that there are a few people that need to work on owning their own truth!

Oftentimes our own ego prevents us from owning our own truth. You must be open and honest with yourself first before you can be open and honest with anyone else. Just like most of the topics we have discussed already, owning your truth is truly a lifestyle change.

Here are a few steps you can do to start living your own truth:

1. Think about where you are currently in your life. Write down all the things you struggle often regardless of what it is, such as health, finances, trust, love etc..

2. Without judging where you are and who you think you own, acknowledge where you are. Take some time and write down who you are today and what you stand for?
3. Talk about your truth. You already know who you are and what you want but allow other people's opinions to dictate your truth. Without judgement, take time to define your truth.

When you think about tranquility most people immediately think about going to being pampered at a spa or the nail salon. However, it's a state of being calm, having a peace of mind and self-care – that most often comes once you start owning your truth. Self-Care is about taking time for yourself to breathe and create peace within you. In those moments is when we can identify what our needs are and not the needs of our families, jobs and business.

N ~ NECESSARY

So far, we have discussed having compassion, being overlooked, working on our mindsets, the process of progress, our life's vision, the importance of taking time out, insurance (both medical and life), and owning your own truth. Now in this final chapter, we are going to discuss why you should dream, imagine, believe, forgive, and the importance of self-care. All of these topics are necessary to your well-being because they all play a role in helping you find completion in your life. Please review the below list:

- It' necessary to dream because we are ambitious creatures who want to aspire to be somebody, rather it's being a coach, a great mom, a great wife, a great entrepreneur you name it.
- It's necessary to imagine the possibilities are endless and know that God made us to move past our struggles and our transgressions.
- It's necessary believe in yourself accept the truth about who you really are without concern of what others may think about you or your situation. Believe in the might God who will not let you fail nor put more on you than you can bare.

- It's necessary to forgive the person who have done us wrong or even ourselves for thinking we allowed it to happen or upset because we did not about what happened.
- Lastly, it's necessary to incorporate self-care practices to maintain our emotional health.

We all have had disappointments, trials, and tribulations at some point in our lives. When you were a child you may not have had both parents, or you may have been adopted. However, you are still alive...therefore, you have already overcome whatever it is that you have went through. The next necessary step is simple: dream, imagine, believe. Now let's talk about dreaming.

To dream is to be daring; it is to revitalize your life. You should evaluate where you are today to understand where you are going tomorrow. You must administer control over your situation and remember to measure your success:

- **D**are – you must have the courage to create the goals you have for yourself and to allow yourself to have big dreams. This is true even for daydreaming because it allows you to see your future. Allow your mind to take you to a place you would have never thought you would be or go, think about the car you always wanted to have, the house you want to get old in, the marriage you've always wanted along with the kids ect.
- **R**evitalize – if you do not revitalize, you will be stuck. There is always a process when it comes to being successful in life rather it a business, a job, being a mom, ect. Remember, you must give yourself a new life.
- **E**valuate – you must always assess where you are in life; remember your past but don't stay stuck to it, reflect on your

future but don't stay focused on it, live for your present, because you must own it.

- **A**dminister – you must remember to manage your life without allowing others to interfere because it's your life and not theirs. You are the only one who can manage or be in control of your situation.
- **M**easure – in addition to all the above, you must have a plan for your life (both personal or business) for what you want to achieve and have a way to measure your success.

Now I want you to create your own meaning for D.R.E.A.M. and reasons why they are important to you. Take your time and really think about it because it will help you to understand what's necessary to YOU. Take the time to create different statements based on what you want to experience:

D:

_____

_____

_____

_____

R:

_____

_____

_____

_____

E:

_____

_____

_____

_____

A:

_____

_____

_____

_____

M:

_____

_____

_____

_____

Let's talk about having an imagination. When I look back over my life, I remember losing my sense of imagination. I forgot how to imagine about living my life in abundance due my illnesses and other trials, and tribulations. At some point of our lives, we all lose it; however, it is necessary to have one. I didn't find my imagination again until I became an entrepreneur; although you don't need to be a business owner to want to imagine how to live your best life. You just need a few action steps to remind you how to imagine. So, I came up with a meaning for I.M.A.G.I.N.E.:

- Introduce (or re-introduce) yourself to your image.
- Multiply your level of importance to yourself.
- Angels are watching over you to ensure that you complete your course.
- Go from being good to great.
- Ignore all the animosity in the world and in your life.
- Negativity has been deleted from your life.
- Energy to complete all tasks.

Now I want to create your own meaning for I.M.A.G.I.N.E. and reasons why they are important to you. Take your time and really think about it because it will help you to understand more of where you are what you want for yourself. Take the time to create different statements based on what you want to experience.

I:

_____

_____

_____

_____

M:

_____

_____

_____

_____

A:

_____

_____

_____

_____

G:

_____

_____

_____

_____

I:

_____

_____

N:

_____

_____

_____

_____

E:

_____

_____

_____

_____

Now that you have created a way to dream again and to imagine living your best life; you must _believe_ it will happen. Our life's circumstances can ruin our belief system to the point that it becomes difficult to believe in ourselves or our abilities. When was the last time you truly believed in yourself without questioning it? After reading different definitions for the word believe, it states: "To accept what is true." Being honest with yourself first _helps_. Below is my interpretation of the word B.E.L.I.E.V.E.:

- **Be** the best that I can be regardless of what my current circumstances dictate. Know that this too shall pass.
- **Eliminate** all the toxic things that has shown up in my life, such as food, fear, procrastination, people etc.
- **Love** everything about who you are, your smile, your stomach, your face, your arms, your personality etc.
- **Incorporate** self-Love by saying your daily affirmations, expressing gratitude, creating a morning ritual, exercise, eat healthy etc.

- Experience new things in your life. You don't know what you don't know so it is important to experiment. i.e., walking by the pond or going to a museum etc.; Do something different!
- Visualize where I am going in this life, such as your next vacation, your house, your car, you next job etc.
- Execute your beliefs by working on them daily.

Now I want you to create your own meaning for B.E.L.I.E.V.E and the reasons why they are important to you. Take your time and really think about it because it will help you to understand more of where you are what you want for yourself. Take the time to create different statements based on what you want to experience:

B:

_____

_____

_____

_____

E:

_____

_____

_____

_____

L:

_____

_____

_____

_____

I:

_____

_____

_____

_____

E:

_____

_____

_____

_____

V:

_____

_____

_____

_____

E:

_____

_____

_____

_____

FORGIVENESS ACTION STEPS

Give yourself Permission to forgive yourself first. Write a letter to yourself. In this letter, you must be brutally honest with what's going on in your thoughts, feelings and emotions; you cannot *release* what you are continuously *reliving*.

- Forgive yourself for not living a healthy lifestyle.
- Forgive yourself for being in that relationship that you finally left.
- Forgive yourself for caring what others don't care about you.
- Forgive yourself for lying to your parents, friends or family.

Remember, forgiveness is not for the other person, it is for you to heal, let go and move one!

COACHING ASSIGNMENT

Think about the things you have encounter over the past few years. Have you had the woulda, coulda, shoulda's thoughts? Great, now is the time to let the past be the past by LETTING IT GO! In the letter, I want you to include the following:

- What that person did to you? Include why you are having a hard time forgiving that person.
- Just because you forgive that person does not mean you are now best friends or must communicate with them. Forgive them without excusing the act because once you forgive it allows you to be at peace.
- Write down how you are going to forgive that person or individuals.

Additional Suggestions:
- Now that you have written a letter to yourself by being brutally honest, now I want you to write a forgiveness statement. This statement should be powerful, and impactful. No matter what you are feeling, when you read the statement hopefully you will feel released, uplifted, and encouraged.
- Next, look for scriptures that speak to your soul and ones that you can meditate on daily.
- Take time to write at least 15 minutes a day by writing down three things you are grateful for daily.
- Write down affirmations that will help you when you need a reminder.
    a. I forgave myself for _____.

b. I have forgiven _____ (if you want you can include their names) because I no longer _____.

- Drink some calming tea (lavender, chamomile ect.), and say your affirmations

After you have written all the information down, you decide what next steps you are going to take. Below are ideas that you can use in order to feel like you have made progress by releasing it:

a. Burn it
b. Throw Darts at it
c. Rip it up and take it to an ocean and allow it to wash away
d. Just tear it up and then toss it in the trash.

Just to reiterate, forgiveness is for you, so you must make a decision on how you will let it go!

Here are few scriptures that I like to use:

Scriptures

1. 1 John 1:9 ESV- If we confess our sins, he is faithful and just to forgives us our sins and to cleanse us from all unrighteousness.
2. Isaiah 43:25-27 ESV- I, I am he who blots out your transgressions for my own sake, and I will not remember your sins, put me in remembrance let us argue together, set forth your case, that you may be proved right. Your first father sinned, and your mediators transgressed against me.
3. Isaiah 1:18 ESV- Come now, let us reason together, says the Lord; though your sins are like scarlet, they shall be as white as snow; though they are red like crimson, they

shall become like wool. If you are willing and obedient, you shall eat the good of the land.
4. Proverbs 19:21 ESV- Many are the plans in the mind of a man, but it is the purposes of the Lord that will stand.
5. St John 10:27 ESV- My sheep hear my voice, and I know them, and they follow me.

It's important that you take the time to write a letter to yourself, create affirmations and include a forgiveness statement because it will help you:

- Create a higher level of self-esteem.
- It will help your love more in your heart.
- It will help to eliminate the stress you have been caring on your shoulders.
- You will begin to smile more due to the amount of peace you feel.
- You will love yourself more because are no longer angry with yourself.
- More importantly, so you can love others and not treat everyone as if they are the problem.

All these things can be a part of your self-care action plan. As women, we are nurturers by Nature! Why, because:

- When someone calls and needs an ear, we listen.
- When someone we know or care about needs something, we try to provide it.
- When our child(ren) are sick, we stay home from work and take care of them.
- When our loved ones are sick, we become their caregiver.
- We cook, we clean, we go to work, we take the kids to their sporting events and we just make things happen.

Through it all, we put ourselves last. These are reasons why Self-Care is so import. As you sit down and think the meaning of self-care for you, I want you dig deep. You don't have to share your answers with anyone I just want to ask that you be honest with yourself. Take a moment and answer these few questions below:

- In your own words, what does wellness and self-care mean to you?
  _____
  _____
  _____
  _____

- What do you currently do for your daily self-care needs?

  How many hours of sleep do you get daily?
  _____
  _____

  How much water do you drink daily?
  _____
  _____

  Are you eating a balanced meal?
  _____
  _____

  How often do you move your bowels?
  _____
  _____

- When was the last time you took 30 minutes to yourself with no social media, no cell phone, no talking to the husband/family? Just you and God or a good book!
- When was the last time dated yourself? Meaning, going to the movies along, take yourself to breakfast, go get your nails and feet done.

85

- When the last time you and your husband or significant other had an entire weekend to yourselves without the kids, you being on your phone all day or social media or conference call?
- When was the last time you felt; love, joy, peace, patience, gentleness, faithfulness, self-control, kindness, and goodness in your life?

How did you feel after answering those question? When I first answered these questions myself, I felt defeated. I felt like I was running myself ragged for no reason because I have so many goals but wasn't getting any of them accomplished. At least that is how I felt after answering the questions; but then I realized, I wanted peace, I wanted more joy, and I wanted to love me more. I also realized that I had to create it for itself because it is not something that can't be given to you. You must love yourself enough to get it done for you because it's what YOU want and what YOU need.

You may have cried while thinking about who you are authentically. We as women wear so many masks: mother, daughter, wife, co-worker, employee, entrepreneur, church sister…often we forget to remove them. So much so that they begin to become a part of us.

After this exercise, you should feel more balance in your life; you should NOT feel guilty about being your authentic self and more importantly, you should realize that you don't owe anyone an explanation. It's necessary!

MOVING FORWARD

To bring these chapters to a close, now is the time to ensure that you have completed each chapter in its entirety. Don't give up too Soon title was created because oftentimes we are close to our destiny, but we give up before we have made it. Each of the steps will help you find more peace, rest your energy, mindset, wellness and tranquility. Now that you have created your own meanings for each chapter, it's time to put them in one place and use it as a foundation to find COMPLETION in your life:

1. How are you going to have more compassion?

   _____

   _____

   _____

2. How are you going to look past being overlooked?

   _____

   _____

   _____

3. What is your current mindset now that you have completed the chapters?

_____

_____

_____

4. What progress have you made sense completing the book?

_____

_____

5. What is in your Life's Vision?

_____

_____

_____

6. Have you made any doctor's appointments lately?

_____

_____

_____

7. How have you taken a Time Out? If so, what did you do?

_____

_____

_____

8. Have you decided on what health or life insurance you are going to have for you or your family?

_____

_____

_____

9. Are you owning your truth?

_____

_____

_____

10. Have you taken the necessary steps to dream, imagine, believe, forgive and have self-care?

_____

_____

_____

Taking the time to really investigate life and remember that the things that you have put in the back of your brain can be difficult to revisit. It will be amazing once you have finally released all the negative energy or a positive gain. Now that you have completed each section, take the time to look at it daily. It will remind you that you are beautifully and wonderfully made and that you are meant for success. Pray over it daily because it will let God know that you are serious about being successful by making the necessary sacrifice your own transformation. Don't just read your affirmations but read them out loud and learn them. The more you speak life over yourself and your situation, the easier it will be to face any obstacles that comes your way.

- Know your self-worth.
- Know your goals.
- Never give up.
- Embrace everything that happens, good, bad or indifferent and acknowledge your feelings instead of running away from them.
- Honor the journey and the struggle because that is what makes you, YOU!

READY SET GO…

I have shared my truth, my trials, tribulations, my pain, my fear and my troubles. I have allowed my illnesses to define my life for far too long until I decided enough was enough. I realized that I was not loving and merely existing. I was not living up to my full potential nor was I striving to live my best life. I had to learn that through my own self-evaluation. I have provided you with the starting point for you to challenge your current self in order to unleash a greater you. Now it's your turn to live your truth. Ready… Set… Go…

Quote:
"Have faith in your heart, passion in your spirit and resilience in your mind and you can do anything. Look beyond your past and elevate your expectations. God will only meet you where you are so in order to grow, you must have expectations that he will do what you ask if it's in his will." (unknown author)

https://www.verywellmind.com/how-to-develop-self-compassion-4158290

https://www.health.harvard.edu/mental-health/4-ways-to-boost-your-self-compassion

https://self-compassion.org/exercise-3-exploring-self-compassion-writing/

https://self-compassion.org/exercise-6-self-compassion-journal/

https://www.dol.gov/general/topic/benefits-leave/fmla

https://www.heart.org/en/healthy-living/healthy-lifestyle/mental-health-and-wellbeing/mental-health-and-heart-health

https://professional.heart.org/professional/ScienceNews/UCM_503383_Heart-Disease-and-Stroke-Statistics---2019-Update.jsp

ABOUT THE AUTHOR

Tinesha Boswell was born and raised in Philadelphia, PA and she is a wife, mother, motivational speaker, Wellness Coach, and author.

Tinesha has a Bachelor of Science in Business Management degree from University of Phoenix. She is also a Certified Wellness Coach, Certified Life Coach, Wife Mentor Coach and is currently studying Nutrition and Aromatherapy.

Tinesha is also the founder of i.P.U.S.H Wellness Coaching and Consulting LLC. Due to her multiple chronic illnesses, she felt the need to help individuals become at peace with their illness by learning how to best deal with their chronic illness.

i.P.U.S.H Wellness mission is to help women PUSH pass their pause by teaching them how to balance their Mind through personal development, their Body with fitness and nutrition, and by creating peace and tranquility in their lives. "When they say I can't, IPUSH to focus my mind, train my body and fight for a healthier life!"

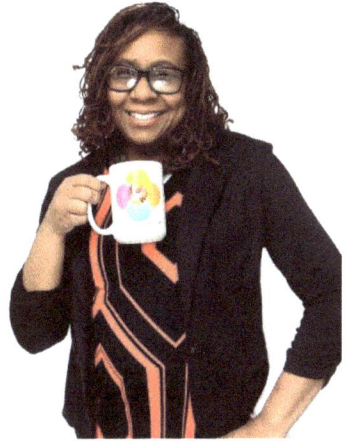

www.ingramcontent.com/pod-product-compliance
Lightning Source LLC
Chambersburg PA
CBHW041300040426
42334CB00028BA/3105